MY ADOLESCENT AS A GIRL CHILD

Tips on how to grow healthy as an adolescent child and live well

BY: A'ISHA SULAYMAN

Table of contents

INTRODUCTION

The adolescent stage of life is characterized by changes in a child's physical, emotional, mental, and social development. However, we initially notice physical changes in order to recognize this stage of life. However, in this case, we'll be talking about "ADOLESCENT AS A GIRL CHILD."

Between childhood and adulthood, there is a time of transformation that may involve physical or psychological development. Teenagers begin between the ages of 10 and 19 years.

Children experience it differently. Just because you start way too early doesn't mean you're not like your childhood friends; you can still hang out with them. Likewise, just because you experience yours later doesn't mean you're weird, make you feel bad about yourself, or cause you to isolate yourself. Be proud of YOU, yourself.

As a parent, you shouldn't worry about your child because they are doing well since things have changed. Instead, you should encourage them, play with them, and be their biggest supporter.

A teenager is defined by the WHO as a person between the ages of 10 and 19. This age group is considered young people by the WHO.

American psychotherapist Erik H. Erikson, who was born in Germany, used the term "Moratorium" to define adolescence in contemporary culture as a time of freedom from adult responsibilities that allows young people to explore several alternatives before deciding on a lifetime job. This theory essentially suggests that one has the opportunity to practice and engage in a wide range of activities during youth before committing to a long-term desire. A youngster should start learning how to take care of himself and their caregiver or parent at this age. Adolescents who are kept away from adult responsibilities for too long may never fully learn how to take care of themselves or the people who depend on them. The co-founder of Microsoft, Bill

Gate, who was developing the company's business plan, is an excellent illustration of a responsible adolescent. But the majority of teenagers play the waiting game, thinking that they won't begin "truly living" until they leave school. This separation from "real life" can be extremely irritating, despite the fact that these years might be helpful in preparing teenagers for their future responsibilities in society
.Many teenagers express themselves in ways that the rest of society finds absurd in order to feel vital and important.

CHAPTER 1
THE CHANGES THAT OCCUR AS WE GROW UP

Girl child puberty: It is obvious that the transition from childhood to adolescence and finally adulthood is a time when the body experiences significant changes, both physically and emotionally. Puberty begins when the hypothalamus, a region of the brain, tells the rest of the body that it is time to start developing adult traits. It transmits these messages via hormones, which in turn trigger the female reproductive system's ovaries to create a variety of additional hormones. Although it may not occur at the same time for everyone, it typically begins between the ages of 8 and 13 and lasts until the age of 15 for girls. It is a process that takes place over several years rather than something that happens immediately.

To better understand:

Hormones, which are organic compounds produced by the body, are in charge of controlling it. The brain and the ovaries produce the hormones that are vital for girls going through puberty.

On either side of the uterus, there are two tiny organs called the ovaries. The ovaries release one or more eggs every month during puberty.

The uterus is a little organ located below the bladder in the lower abdomen. This is where the body develops during pregnancy.

Fallopian tubes are structures with a tube shape that connect the ovaries to the uterus. They transport the egg that the ovaries have released to the uterus.

Progesterone and estrogen are the hormones produced in the ovaries. The majority of the physical changes that occur during puberty are caused by them.

PHYSICAL CHANGES: CHANGES

The breasts will initially begin to form. Just a tiny amount of swelling under the nipple was the first sign.

While the waist gets smaller and there is more fat around the stomach and buttocks, the hips and thighs are growing more curves and becoming a little wider. Gaining additional weight during this time is typical and healthy. There is no such thing as "normal" at this period because it develops differently for each person. Everybody develops their own individual size and shape.

Hair is growing in the pubic region, beneath the arms, and on the legs.

a rise in height. This 'growth spurt' occurs quickly. After starting their menstrual cycle, girls often cease growing taller in around 2 years.

At this period, your genes—the informational code you acquired from your parents—will determine a number of factors, including your height, weight, breast size, and even how much hair you have on your body.

Vulvar discharge is a light to moderate quantity of vaginal discharge that starts

between 6 and 12 months before the first period. It is a typical reaction to the body's rising levels of the estrogen hormone.
MENSTRUATION: It can happen at any time, but it often begins between two to three years of the development of the breast buds.
Other alterations consist of:
more sweating
emergence of acne (pimples)
When one first becomes attracted to someone romantically or sexually, this is called attraction
MOTIVATING EMOTIONS
Hormones don't just address bodily changes. The same estrogen hormones that induce physical changes in females also have an impact on how they feel emotionally, or how they feel about themselves. This time period can be emotionally turbulent. You could
Be apprehensive about the changes one minute and enthusiastic about them the next.

Uncomfortable or perplexed
Laughter one second, tears the next
Fight on the same day while getting along
with your family and friends.
Feel constantly enraged and hungry
SELF-ADMIRATION TO ADOLESCENT
AND PARENT: Feel like a child one day and
like a grownup the next
Please, always be yourself. Speak your mind
and surround yourself with friendly and
decent people. Take pride in who you are.
Spend your time carefully and strive to
always offer value to yourself.
Nobody can be you; you are who you are.
You are special.
Never permit negativity or self neglect of
any kind.
Avoid being envious of your friends.
Take compliments and express them to
others.
keep up a good example
Treat yourself and those around you with
kindness.

Your buddy's stature is excellent and she receives compliments frequently; don't ignore it. Likewise, if your friend is big, don't body shame her. If she is skinny, don't make fun of her self-esteem. You are different from your friend because of the gene you acquired from your parents.
You don't need to change who you are for anyone because you are beautiful just the way you are. Parent: Support them in their choices while also letting them discover things on their own, make mistakes, and learn from them so they can come to terms with who they are and their responsibilities. Be a good listener to them so they can always come to you instead of picking up every negative behavior in society or their friends, be a kind guide who gives and shows them love and care since they are at a stage where they need it all. They need you more than they need their nanny and friends. Be their best friends.

CHAPTER 2

PERIOD

Period is the month to month vaginal draining that happens to each lady of development age as a feature of month to month cycle. It happens when a lady is of pubescence and physically dynamic to replicate, it happens when there is an arrival of egg from the ovaries to the uterus hanging tight for preparation y the sperm of a man however no treatment happen, such egg is shed from the uterus lining what somewhat contains blood and mostly tissue from the uterus. It normally lasts 3-7days. There are a few different side effects before the start of the draining which we call PREMENSTRUAL SYNDROME which are:

Stomach or pelvic spasm

Lower back torment

Swelling or sore bosom

Food desires

Temperament swings and touchiness

Cerebral pain and exhaustion

MENSTRUAL CYCLE: It starts with the principal day of your period and begins once more when the following time frame starts. The month to month cycle lasts between 24-38days. It is counted from the principal day of your period up to the main day of the following one which stands as the quantity of days for the cycle. The chemicals estrogen and progesterone are the one working and causing changes in the monthly cycle. After the arrival of ova(egg) into the uterus the progesterone chemical begin to get ready for pregnancy which occurs in the event that there is preparation from the sperm cell yet in the event that there is none the lining of the uterus is shed as MENSTRUATION

OVULATION: The arrival of egg from the ovary into the uterus planning for treatment by a sperm cell. A lady is probably going to get pregnant in the event that she engages in sexual relations without conception prevention during this period which is probably going to be during the 3days previously and up to the day of ovulation (assuming the sperm cell is now set up and prepared to treat the egg when it is delivered). A man's sperm cell can satisfy 3-5days in a lady's regenerative organ, yet a lady's egg lives for only 12-24hrs after ovulation.

Every lady cycle length might be unique and the time among ovulation and when the following time frame start can be remotely close to seven days to over about fourteen days

The most effective method to be aware assuming you ovulating

A couple of days before ovulation the vaginal bodily fluid or release changes and becomes more dangerous and clear. A few ladies feel minor squeezing on one side of their pelvic region when they ovulate.
NOTE
Not many years after the first period,menstrual periods longer than 38days are normal. Young ladies normally get more standard cycles in no less than three years of beginning

In your 20's and 30's, your cycles are normally standard and can endure somewhere in the range of 24-38days. Following

Standard following assists with knowing when you ovulate, when you are liable to get pregnant and when to anticipate your next period. Not customary, following can assist share issues with specialists or medical attendants.

STEP BY STEP INSTRUCTIONS TO TRACK

By denoting the day you start your period on a calendar. Following a couple of months you can check whether it is standard or not. You can likewise follow by checking your PMS side effects, for example, squeezing, cerebral pain, irritability, distracted, bulging or bosom delicacy.

While the draining happened was it before or later than anticipated?

Period side effects: Was there torment/draining that you missed everyday schedule

How long does it last? More limited or longer than the prior month.

PERIOD SYMPTOMS

Bosom delicacy

Skin break out

Squeezing in the lower mid-region and back

More craving

Rest issue

State of mind swings

Swelling

MENSTRUAL CYCLE PATTERN

An egg is ready and is delivered by one of your ovaries. This is called ovulation

Long before ovulation, estrogen increments and makes your body foster a thick uterine covering that is made of blood and tissue. This is the manner by which the uterus prepare for conceivable pregnancy

On the off chance that you have intercourse close to this time and the egg is prepared by sperm, it will go to the uterus and append itself to the uterine wall. Then leisurely form into a child.

On the off chance that the egg isn't prepared, it does it append to the mass of the uterus. The uterus needn't bother with the additional tissue lining, so it shed it. Assuming that the blood, tissue and unfertilized egg leave the uterus, going through the vagina on the exit plan the body is PERIOD

MENSTRUAL BLOOD

Blood is a liquid connective tissue that contains plasma, platelets and Platelets. It courses all through the body conveying oxygen and supplements to different cells and tissue. It makes up 8% of our body weight. A typical grown-up has around 5-6litres.

Blood contains four parts which are plasma (55%), Erythrocytes (RBC), Leukocytes (WBC) and Platelets. Plasma gives water, salts, lipids and chemicals. It is uniquely wealthy in protein ALBUMIN. The fundamental protein, immunoglobulin, coagulating elements and fibrinogen.

Plasma performs a few capabilities, for example,
Moving platelets and supplements
Controlling the body water and mineral salts
Inundating tissues
Giving safeguard against contamination and
Coagulating blood
Egg whites: the egg whites contained in plasma keeps the blood from losing an excess of water and consistency as it's movement through the thin water porous veins (vessels). Egg whites transport different blood parts and supplements.
IMMUNOGLOBULIN: additionally contained in plasma are antibodies that alongside WBC assume a significant part I battling against microbes.
Coagulation FACTORS: in mix with platelets controls drain.
WBC: resistance and protection system. They cleanse and shield the body from disease. When a contamination is distinguished in any piece of the body, the WBC moves in and battles.

RBC: A drop of blood the size of a pin head contains roughly 5m RBC. They get their red tone from an iron containing protein called Hemoglobin. RBC makes up between 37-44% of the volume of blood in ladies. It conveys oxygen all through the body. PLATELETS/THROMBOCYTES: it is a particular platelet delivered from bone marrow. It becomes possibly the most important factor when there is drain (dying) . It helps in thickening and coagulation of blood. Helps in coagulation during cut or wound.

Capability of blood:

Gives oxygen to the cells.

Transport chemicals and supplement Homeostasis i.e helps in keeping up with the inside internal heat level by engrossing or delivering heat.

Blood coagulating at the site of injury.

Transport of waste to the kidney and liver.

Safeguard the body against microbes.

PACK CELL VOLUME(PCV)

It is a straightforward blood test. It is a test accomplished for a call complete body count (CBC), estimating the extent of RBC in the blood. Lower than ordinary measure of blood in the body can show:
Inadequate stockpile of solid RBC(anemia).
A bigger number is WBC due to long haul disease, contamination or a WBC issue called Leukemia/LYMPHOMA.
Nutrient or mineral insufficiency.
Ongoing or long haul blood misfortune.
Higher than typical can show:
Drying out
Lung or coronary illness
Having a hematocrit meaning PCV test done is to know the level of blood volume in one's body which is made out of RBC which range from age to sex yet for female grown-up 18 over 35-47 (University of Iowa Diagnostic Laboratory) and for youngsters 17 and more youthful 34-44 (University of Iowa Diagnostic Laboratory). Having a low degree of protein to give Hemoglobin causes Anemia (iron lack). Side effects include:

Weariness

Dazedness

Windedness

Heart palpitations

Reasons for low RBC count include:

Low degree of iron in the body

Persistent kidney sickness

Blood misfortune

Lack of healthy sustenance

NOTE: Blood misfortune can come in for an adolescent that has begun to get her period and has a weighty stream. An adolescent can have low RBC count because of a weighty stream which makes it motivation to have an iron rich protein. WE WILL TALK ABOUT DIET IN NEXT CHAPTER.

For more comprehension of how low RBC include can happen in a adolescent due to heavy feminine stream: Read underneath;

After a weighty period, there is loss of some iron which is in a course of getting reestablished then another feminine cycle happen and there is stream again a weighty one and it proceeds with like that without getting completely or enough reclamation or recuperated from the past misfortune and afterward misfortune and afterward misfortune.

Then, an adolescent falls into having a low RBC count. Justification for why a developing adolescent or passed on say female or ladies in everyday requirements to have an iron rich eating routine all time.

CHAPTER 3

NUTRITION

As an adolescent going through actual changes and advancement and furthermore mental and close to home changes remembering chemicals and changes for hormonal emission and levels. There will be a need for extra admission of energy distraught other supplements for appropriate development and improvement.

NUTRITIONAL REQUIREMENTS

ENERGY: Calories prerequisites is assessed in kcal shifting in age and sex and adding an additional consumptions with everyday exercises. The greatest utilization of calories for female yells is assessed around 2500kcal in the menarche period and declines dynamically to 2200kcal after that.

PROTEIN: It ordinarily agrees with the greatest energy prerequisites during pubertal spray and they might be assessed around 12-15 of the complete calories of females.

Age	Total daily proteins	Calories
11-14	0.29	14.0
15-19	0.28	12.9
20-24	0.27	12.9

Yet, it is considered to have an expansion in incentive for adolescents that work out or that live in "willful prohibitive eating regimens" as a reason for anorexia nervosa. FAT: In an eating routine fat acts as a concentrated wellspring of energy toons fat dissolvable nutrients and as a hotspot for fundamental unsaturated fats, giving around 30% of the prerequisites. For the development of a young adult such a lot of energy is required that without fat the eating routine will become tacky. In any case, then again, high fat tidbits and a stationery way of life which is a typical way of behaving among adolescents is answerable for corpulence and arteriosclerosis. This is an extraordinary advantage to diminish the level of complete fats and immersed fats. SUGARS: The fundamental wellspring of energy for young adults typically contributes 55%of everyday calorie admission. The monosaccharides glucose and fructose which are available in leafy foods are specialists of "sweet" sugar. Fructose utilization found in sodas syrup is answerable for the expanded weight. Disaccharide are sucrose, lactose and maltose are available in most adjusted diet that incorporates vegetable, grains and milk MINERALS: Most significant minerals during young adulthood incorporate basically calcium, iron and zinc. Prohibitive eating regimens and game contests impact bone mineralization causing osteoporosis, osteopenia, pubertal postponement.

Complete body calcium, 97% of it is allotted into weight and in extent , it increments emphatically during adolescent development and advancement. This, a typical day to day admission of 1200mg of calcium is suggested relying upon the need(based on proactive tasks) of the adolescent .

In iron, it prerequisites increases with the development of bulk, blood volume and respiratory limit adjacent to menstrual loss of iron in blood. Iron substance for food likewise goes from 4-6mg or 1000kcal. Thus, young adults that bleed and don't get the aggregate sum of iron required, which is determined to be around 15-18mg each day during pubertal spray. Need for mineral supplementation will rely upon the assortment and nature of diet, mostly during pubertal spray.
VITAMIN: The prerequisite expands in adolescence because of expanded anabolism and vigorous use. Need for vitamin A,B,C and D are continuously higher during adolescence with cell separation and bone mineralization. Everyday admission of

natural product, vegetable, milk and cereals gives the necessary nutrient.

SOUND NUTRITION

PROTEIN: It is crafted by development and fundamental advancement of organs as well as tissue recovery. Creature and vegetable protein sources incorporate meat, fish, chicken, milk, soy, grains and seeds, beans and cereal which assists with providing 20-25% of the all out calories in an everyday eating regimen.

STARCHES: It gives lively capability and assurance digestion and internal heat level. They are tracked down in grains, rice, wheat, oats, flour, bread and pasta.

LIPIDS: They have fundamental caloric capability that is completed by immersed and non soaked fat, presents in oils, soybeans, spreads, magazines, fat, greases, hotdogs, cream, sauce, fries and mayonnaise.

VITAMIN AND MINERALS: Functions of controlling or keeping up with the musicality of the cell and enzymatic reaction. Principal sources are vegetables, entire oats, milk, seed, meat, eggs and grains

Water, juices, coconut milk and different wellsprings of fluids ought to be drunk on normal 4-6 glasses per day, however on blistering days, after exercise and game exercises in the sun it ought to be expanded to 6-8glasses.

Liquor and invigorating beverages also as anabolic steroids are not prudent.

During the development stage, milk which is the primary wellsprings of calcium,protein protein and nutrient ought to be important for day to day diet with 2-3 glasses per day and some part of journal items, for example, yogurt, cheddar, frozen yogurt and pudding ought to be added.

However, in controlling weight, whole milk ought to be supplanted low fat or fat free milk

NOTE: NO particular eating regimen for all adolescents. It is sufficient as per development and phases of adolescence, everyday exercises and way of life (Einstein et al)

Nourishing lack and unfortunate dietary pattern in immaturity can have a drawn out results including postponed sexual development, loss of conclusive grown-up level, osteoporosis and heftiness. For veggie lovers, adolescent gamble incorporates absence of iodine, vitamin B12 and D and fundamental unsaturated fats (R. Wahl).

GUIDE TO HELP YOU CHOOSE AND KNOW THE VALUE OF WHAT TO EAT

Bread, grain and cereals are carbs that give energy to mind and muscle. Likewise an amazing wellspring of fiber and vitamin B. Without enough starches you feel drained and broken down.

Leafy foods have parcels of nutrients and minerals that assist with supporting an invulnerable framework and hold one back from becoming ill. Likewise significant for sound skin and eyes.

Meat, fish, egg, nuts and vegetables are great wellsprings of iron and protein and as a female adolescent you really want sufficient iron in light of the fact that as you bleed you lose iron and you will generally have weakness. Protein is required for development, to keep muscle solid, decline in it might prompt hindered level and weight. Fish is great for mind, eye and skin and for veggie lovers that don't eat meat there are alternate ways of meeting your iron e.g lentils, nuts and seeds, and prepared beans.

Journal food like milk, cheddar and yogurt assists with building bones and teeth and keeps your heart, muscles and nerves working appropriately.

A lot of fat and oil can bring about gaining weight. Other high fat food like chocolate, chips, cakes and seared food sources can expand your weight without giving the body numerous supplements.

Liquid is an additionally significant piece of diet. It assists with keeping you hydrated and furthermore assists with forestalling blockage.

CHAPTER 4
STRESS/OVERWORK ON GROWTH OF AN ADOLESCENT GIRL

Growing up there are a parcel of exercises that channel one genuinely and sincerely, for example, shuffling after school exercises, sport practice, schoolwork, apprenticeship program among others. Prompting some impact like absence of sufficient rest, absence of focus in school and different exercises, prompting normal or terrible showing. However it is realized a prudent that additional roundabout exercises like game or learning of one exchange and being a disciple helps adolescent to acquire important experience and a few other required abilities, makes them more capable and be time cognizant and furthermore in cash the executives however at that point there ought as far as possible and observe a straightforward guideline, for, having opportunity and willpower to rest and not revel in exercises, feed well, rest proficiently and don't work in a perilous climate.

Exhausting/long haul pressure can add to physical and psychological well-being issues, broadened pressure can cause hypertension, debilitate the resistant framework and add to sickness like heftiness and coronary illness. Furthermore, some psychological well-being issue such as nervousness distraught melancholy

Indications of stress in adolescent should be visible in manners like:
Peevishness and outrage
Changes in conduct
Inconvenience dozing
Disregarding liability
Change in eating habits.

In young adult it tends to be overseen and hold in line by:
Resting soundly.
Work out.
Work it out with grown-ups.
Investing energy out.
Working it out as a type of articulation.

CHAPTER 5
HEALTHY DIET + HEALTHY LIFESTYLE = HEALTHY LIVING

Healthy eating routine can be obstructed and accomplished on such countless factors, for example,

In view of accessibility, convenience and time as opposed to food esteem.

Peer bunch, broad communications and self-perception commitment or impact

Individual degree of confidence

Practicing good eating habits

Food helps in development and living in adolescent in such countless ways, for example,

Accomplishing quick development and full development potential.

Helps in opportune sexual development.

A solid eating regimen with sufficient number of calcium statements in the bone aids in accomplishing legitimate bone strength.

Having a solid eating routine sets the vibe for a lifetime of smart dieting which assists with saving corpulence, osteoporosis and diabetes sometime down the road.
Laying out a sound living eating routine with a legitimate measure of lack of iron assists with forestalling iron frailty in an adolescent young lady.
Little kids who have the propensity for skipping feasts and benefiting from tidbits or cheap food joints with food low in calories and other necessary supplements do not develop well and become hindered in development. Such adolescent young ladies are probably going to endure weakness on account of unfortunate utilization or iron rich food varieties and furthermore because of worm perversion and regular contamination.

Good dieting propensity for young adult young lady ought to incorporate the accompanying nutrition type:
A lot of leafy foods.

Appropriate amount of rice and different cereals, potatoes, noodles and pasta.
A few milk and journal items like yogurt and cheddar.
Some meat, fish, poultry egg and additionally nuts and vegetables.
Likewise pick food that is low in salts.
Limit food that contains parcel of sugar and fats
"An individual generally speaking well-being is more than a shortfall of infection. It is a condition of complete physical, mental and social prosperity. It is a vital aspect for carrying on with a useful and fulfilling way of life"

Sound way of life propensity for young adult include:
Work out: At Least an adolescent ought to be truly exercised for 60 mins in a day, stay away from a stationary way of life.
Develop the propensity for having nutritious dinner.
Keep a solid weight.

Get sufficient rest: try not to rest so
particularly late as it has an impact on your
capacity to focus and get along nicely at
school.
Try not to pay attention to noisy music.
The most effective method to deal with
emotional well-being as a young adult:
Learn ways of overseeing pressure as this
assists with remaining even headed and
have the option to work in distressing
circumstances and hold outrage under
control.
Review and make an honest effort to do well
in school.
A sound connection with parents goes far as
this can likewise assist in troublesome times
as they fill in as shoulder to rest on more
than companions as they need the best for
you.
Have a legitimate harmony between school,
work and public activity, try not to exhaust
and don't invest an excess of energy via
virtual entertainment or hanging with
companions.

Try not to attempt to take on something over the top. Do the main ones and give your best 100 percent. Workaholic behavior can prompt pressure, disappointment or depletion.

EMOTIONAL HEALTH: your inclination Focus on your sentiments and states of mind. Try not to constantly expect your awful thoughts as feelings are simply an aspect of growing up. Assuming you are stressed over something, request help.

Feel free to request help.

Acknowledge yourself: Don't peer down on yourself and what you can do, don't permit somebody's meaning to get to you, forever be caring and decent, take on your likes,dream and despise you. Carry on with your life at the best. Take on great and solid carrying on with your way of life.

BEHAVIORAL HEALTH

Stay away from savagery

Stay away from substance use or misuse

Practice forbearance (no sex) or safe sex.